## OUR DAILY HEALTHCARE.

Health care refers to the maintenance and improvement of a person's physical and mental well-being through the prevention, diagnosis, treatment, and management of illness and injury. Health care typically involves a wide range of professionals, including doctors, nurses, pharmacists, therapists, and other healthcare providers who work together to provide medical care to patients.

Health care can be provided in a variety of settings, including hospitals, clinics, nursing homes, and home care settings. It can also include a range of services, such as primary care, specialized medical care, preventive care, rehabilitation, and palliative care.

In many countries, access to healthcare is considered a basic human right, and governments are responsible for providing healthcare services to their citizens. The provision of healthcare services can be funded through a variety of sources, such as government programs, private insurance, or out-of-pocket payments.

**HOW TO improve our daily health care**

---

There are several ways to improve your daily health care routine:

1. Get enough sleep: Getting enough sleep is essential for good health. Aim for at least 7-8 hours of sleep each night.

2. Eat a healthy diet: Eating a balanced diet that includes plenty of fruits, vegetables, whole grains, lean proteins, and healthy fats can help keep your body healthy.

3. Exercise regularly: Regular exercise can help keep your body and mind healthy. Aim for at least 30 minutes of moderate exercise, such as walking, cycling, or swimming, most days of the week.

4. Practice good hygiene: Good hygiene habits, such as washing your hands regularly, brushing your teeth twice a day, and showering regularly, can help prevent the spread of germs and keep you healthy.

5. Get regular check-ups: Regular check-ups with your healthcare provider can help detect and treat health problems early.

6. Manage stress: Stress can have a negative impact on your health. Practice stress-management techniques, such as meditation, deep breathing, or yoga, to help reduce stress.

7. Limit alcohol and tobacco use: Limiting your alcohol and tobacco use can help reduce your risk of developing many health problems, such as heart disease, cancer, and respiratory problems.

By incorporating these habits into your daily routine, you can improve
your overall health and well-being.

## Health development and care

Health development and care refer to the ongoing process of improving health outcomes and providing care to individuals and communities. It involves a range of activities, including health promotion, disease prevention, diagnosis, treatment, rehabilitation, and palliative care.

Health development aims to improve the health of individuals and communities by addressing the underlying social, economic, and environmental factors that influence health. This includes activities such as improving access to clean water and sanitation, promoting healthy behaviors such as exercise and healthy eating, and reducing social and economic inequalities that can lead to poor health outcomes.

Health care, on the other hand, focuses on the delivery of medical services to individuals. It includes a range of services, such as primary care, specialized medical care, preventive care, rehabilitation, and palliative care. Health care providers work together to diagnose and treat illness and injury, manage chronic conditions, and provide care and support to individuals and families.

Both health development and care are essential components of a comprehensive health system. By focusing on both prevention and treatment, health systems can improve health outcomes, reduce healthcare costs, and promote overall well-being.

**Important activities we should do daily in other to maintain a good health standard**

Maintaining a good health standard involves several daily activities that can improve your physical, mental, and emotional well-being. Here are some important activities that you should aim to do daily:

1. Eat a balanced diet: A balanced diet that includes plenty of fruits, vegetables, whole grains, lean proteins, and healthy fats can help keep your body healthy.

2. Exercise regularly: Regular exercise can help keep your body and mind healthy. Aim for at least 30 minutes of moderate exercise, such as walking, cycling, or swimming, most days of the week.

3. Get enough sleep: Getting enough sleep is essential for good health. Aim for at least 7-8 hours of sleep each night.

4. Practice good hygiene: Good hygiene habits, such as washing your hands regularly, brushing your teeth twice a day, and showering regularly, can help prevent the spread of germs and keep you healthy.

5. Stay hydrated: Drinking plenty of water each day can help keep your body hydrated and functioning properly.

6. Manage stress: Stress can have a negative impact on your health. Practice stress-management techniques, such as meditation, deep breathing, or yoga, to help reduce stress.

7. Limit alcohol and tobacco use: Limiting your alcohol and tobacco use can help reduce your risk of developing many health problems, such as heart disease, cancer, and respiratory problems.

8. Stay socially connected: Maintaining social connections with friends and family can help improve your mental and emotional well-being.

By incorporating these daily activities into your routine, you can improve your overall health and well-being.

**The effects of not doing all these activities or doing the opposite side**

Not doing the activities listed above, or doing the opposite of them, can have negative effects on your health. Here are some examples:

1. Lack of sleep: Not getting enough sleep can lead to fatigue, irritability, and difficulty concentrating. Chronic sleep deprivation has also been linked to an increased risk of obesity, diabetes, and cardiovascular disease.

2. Lack of exercise: Not getting enough exercise can lead to weight gain, muscle weakness, and poor cardiovascular health. It can also increase the risk of chronic diseases such as diabetes, heart disease, and cancer.

3. Poor diet: A poor diet that is high in processed foods, sugary drinks, and saturated and trans fats can lead to weight gain, high cholesterol, and increased risk of chronic diseases such as diabetes, heart disease, and cancer.

4. Dehydration: Not drinking enough water can lead to dehydration, which can cause fatigue, headaches, and dizziness. Chronic dehydration can also lead to kidney problems and urinary tract infections.

5. Chronic stress: Chronic stress can lead to anxiety, depression, and other mental health problems. It can also increase the risk of chronic diseases such as heart disease, diabetes, and autoimmune disorders.

6. Poor hygiene: Poor hygiene habits can increase the risk of infectious diseases such as colds, flu, and COVID-19.

In summary, not doing the activities listed above or doing the opposite of them can have negative effects on your physical and mental health, and increase the risk of chronic diseases.

## IMPORTANCE OF daily social health care and life span improvement

Daily social health care can have a significant impact on individuals' overall health and well-being, especially as they age. Social health care encompasses a wide range of activities and services that aim to improve people's social connectedness, access to resources, and overall quality of life. Some examples of daily social health care activities might include:

- Participating in social clubs or organizations
- Engaging in regular physical activity
- Spending time with friends and family
- Volunteering or giving back to the community
- Participating in educational activities

Research has shown that social isolation and loneliness can have negative impacts on both physical and mental health, including increased risk of chronic illnesses, depression, and cognitive decline. Conversely, having strong social connections can improve overall health outcomes and increase life expectancy.

In addition to the benefits for individuals, daily social health care can also have broader impacts on society as a whole. By promoting social connectedness and community engagement, social health care can help to reduce healthcare costs, improve public health outcomes, and strengthen social cohesion.

Overall, daily social health care is crucial for improving individuals' quality of life and promoting healthy aging, and should be considered an important component of any comprehensive healthcare

## SYSTEM.**CONCLUSION ON SOCIAL HEALTH CARE**

In conclusion, social health care is an essential component of healthcare systems, especially for promoting healthy aging and improving overall health outcomes. Social isolation and loneliness can have negative impacts on physical and mental health, and social health care programs can help to address these issues by providing opportunities for social connectedness and community engagement. Community-based organizations, technology, intergenerational connections, and social prescribing can all play a role in promoting social health care. The impact of social health care programs extends beyond individuals to include broader societal benefits such as reduced healthcare costs, improved public health outcomes, and strengthened social cohesion. Addressing social determinants of health and promoting cultural competence in social health care services are also important considerations. Overall, social health care is a vital aspect of healthcare systems that should be prioritized in efforts to promote health and well-being.

## BRANCHES OF HEALTH CARE

Healthcare is a broad field that encompasses a wide range of specialties and sub-specialties. Some of the main branches of healthcare include:

1. Primary Care: This is the first point of contact for patients seeking medical attention. Primary care providers include family physicians, pediatricians, and general practitioners who provide preventive care, diagnose and treat common illnesses, and manage chronic conditions.

2. Internal Medicine: This branch of healthcare focuses on the prevention, diagnosis, and treatment of adult diseases. Internal medicine physicians, also known as internists, specialize in the care of adults and often have expertise in managing complex medical conditions.

3. Pediatrics: This branch of healthcare focuses on the health and well-being of infants, children, and adolescents. Pediatricians are trained to diagnose and treat a wide range of childhood illnesses and to provide preventive care, including vaccinations.

4. Obstetrics and Gynecology: This branch of healthcare focuses on the health of women throughout their lives, including pregnancy, childbirth, and menopause. Obstetricians and gynecologists provide preventive care, diagnosis and treatment of gynecological conditions, and care during pregnancy and childbirth.

5. Surgery: This branch of healthcare involves the use of surgical procedures to diagnose and treat medical conditions. Surgeons may specialize in a particular area of the body or a specific type of surgery, such as cardiovascular surgery or neurosurgery.

6. Psychiatry: This branch of healthcare focuses on the diagnosis and treatment of mental health disorders, including depression, anxiety, and schizophrenia. Psychiatrists may use medication, therapy, or a combination of both to treat their patients.

7. Rehabilitation: This branch of healthcare focuses on helping patients recover from injury or illness and regain function and independence. Rehabilitation specialists, such as physical therapists and occupational therapists, work with patients to develop treatment plans that may include exercise, therapy, and assistive devices.

8. Emergency Medicine: This branch of healthcare involves the treatment of patients who require immediate medical attention due to injury or illness. Emergency medicine physicians are trained to quickly diagnose and treat a wide range of medical emergencies, from heart attacks to severe injuries.

9. Radiology: This branch of healthcare involves the use of medical imaging technologies, such as X-rays, CT scans, and MRI scans, to diagnose and treat medical conditions. Radiologists are trained to interpret these imaging studies and provide guidance to other healthcare providers based on the results.

There are many other branches of healthcare, including nursing, dentistry, optometry, and more. Each of these specialties plays a crucial role in ensuring that patients receive the best possible care for their specific needs.

## PRIMARY CARE AND INTERNAL DIAGNOSIS AND ITS EFFECTS AND IMPACT

Primary care and internal medicine are two important branches of healthcare that focus on the prevention, diagnosis, and treatment of medical conditions. Here are some of their effects and impacts:

Primary Care:
- Primary care providers are often the first point of contact for patients seeking medical attention. They provide preventive care, diagnose and treat common illnesses, and manage chronic conditions.
- Primary care providers have a significant impact on patient outcomes, including reducing hospitalizations, improving patient satisfaction, and increasing the likelihood of early diagnosis and treatment of medical conditions.
- Primary care providers play a crucial role in promoting health and wellness in their patients through education and counseling on topics such as diet, exercise, and smoking cessation.
- Access to primary care has been shown to reduce healthcare costs by reducing the need for hospitalizations and emergency room visits.

Internal Medicine:
- Internal medicine physicians specialize in the care of adults and often have expertise in managing complex medical conditions.
- Internal medicine physicians play a crucial role in the diagnosis and treatment of chronic medical conditions, such as diabetes, heart disease, and hypertension, which are major contributors to morbidity and mortality.
- Internal medicine physicians work closely with other healthcare providers to coordinate care for patients with complex medical needs, including those with multiple chronic conditions.

- Internal medicine physicians also play a key role in preventive care, including screening for cancer and other diseases, and providing vaccinations and other preventive interventions.

Overall, primary care and internal medicine are critical components of the healthcare system, providing patients with access to preventive care, diagnosis and treatment of medical conditions, and coordination of care for those with complex medical needs. By promoting health and wellness, preventing and managing chronic conditions, and providing timely and appropriate care, primary care and internal medicine physicians can have a significant impact on patient outcomes and healthcare costs.

## OTHER branches and its effects and impact

---

Here are further explanations of the branches of healthcare you mentioned, along with their effects and impacts:

Pediatrics:
- Pediatrics is the branch of healthcare that focuses on the health and well-being of infants, children, and adolescents.
- Pediatricians are trained to diagnose and treat a wide range of childhood illnesses and to provide preventive care, including vaccinations.
- The impact of pediatric care can be seen in the reduction of infant mortality rates, improved child health outcomes, and the prevention of long-term health problems through early intervention and prevention.
- Pediatricians also play a crucial role in promoting healthy development and providing support to families through counseling and education.


Obstetrics and Gynecology:
- Obstetrics and gynecology (OB/GYN) is the branch of healthcare that focuses on the health of women throughout their lives, including pregnancy, childbirth, and menopause.

- OB/GYNs provide preventive care, diagnosis and treatment of gynecological conditions, and care during pregnancy and childbirth.
- The impact of OB/GYN care can be seen in the reduction of maternal and infant mortality rates, improved reproductive health outcomes, and the prevention and early detection of gynecological cancers.
- OB/GYNs also play a crucial role in promoting sexual and reproductive health through education and counseling.

Rehabilitation:
- Rehabilitation is the branch of healthcare that focuses on helping patients recover from injury or illness and regain function and independence.
- Rehabilitation specialists, such as physical therapists and occupational therapists, work with patients to develop treatment plans that may include exercise, therapy, and assistive devices.
- The impact of rehabilitation can be seen in the improvement of patients' quality of life, increased independence, and the prevention of long-term disability.
- Rehabilitation also plays a crucial role in improving patient outcomes after surgery or other medical procedures.

Emergency Medicine:
- Emergency medicine is the branch of healthcare that involves the treatment of patients who require immediate medical attention due to injury or illness.
- Emergency medicine physicians are trained to quickly diagnose and treat a wide range of medical emergencies, from heart attacks to severe injuries.
- The impact of emergency medicine can be seen in the reduction of morbidity and mortality from acute medical conditions, improved patient outcomes, and the prevention of long-term disability.

- Emergency medicine also plays a crucial role in disaster response and preparedness.


Radiology:
- Radiology is the branch of healthcare that involves the use of medical imaging technologies, such as X-rays, CT scans, and MRI scans, to diagnose and treat medical conditions.
- Radiologists are trained to interpret these imaging studies and provide guidance to other healthcare providers based on the results.
- The impact of radiology can be seen in the early detection and diagnosis of medical conditions, improved patient outcomes, and the ability to guide medical interventions, such as surgery or radiation therapy.
- Radiology also plays a crucial role in cancer screening and prevention, as well as in the management of chronic medical conditions.

## HEALTH CARE TOPICS AND DEFINITION

**Sure, here is a brief explanation of each of the topics:**

1. Health care system - A network of organizations, people, and resources that deliver health care services to meet the health needs of a specific population.

2. Health care policy - The set of laws, regulations, and guidelines that govern the organization, financing, and delivery of health care services.

3. Health care reform - The process of changing and improving the health care system to address deficiencies in access, quality, and affordability.

4. Health care disparities - Differences in health outcomes and access to health care services between different populations, often related to social determinants of health such as race, ethnicity, income, and geography.

5. Health care access - The ability of individuals to obtain needed health care services, often influenced by factors such as insurance coverage, affordability, and geographic proximity.

6. Health care delivery - The process of providing health care services to individuals, including diagnosis, treatment, and management of health conditions.

7. Health care quality - The degree to which health care services meet established standards of safety, effectiveness, and patient-centeredness.

8. Health insurance - A contract between an individual and an insurance company that provides coverage for health care services.

9. Medicare - A federal health insurance program primarily for people aged 65 and older, as well as some younger individuals with disabilities or certain health conditions.

10. Medicaid - A joint federal-state program that provides health insurance coverage for eligible low-income individuals and families.

11. Affordable Care Act - A federal law enacted in 2010 that expanded access to health insurance coverage and implemented various reforms to the health care system.

12. Electronic health records - Digital records of patients' health information that can be shared between health care providers to improve care coordination and quality.

13. Health care costs - The total expenses associated with providing and receiving health care services, including costs for insurance, treatment, and medication.

14. Health care financing - The methods by which health care services are paid for, including insurance, government programs, and out-of-pocket payments.

15. Health care workforce - The individuals who provide health care services, including physicians, nurses, therapists, and other health care professionals.

16. Health care management - The administration and oversight of health care organizations, including hospitals, clinics, and other health care facilities.

**17**. Health care innovation - The development and implementation of new and improved health care technologies, treatments, and delivery models.

18. Health care technology - The tools and devices used to diagnose, treat, and manage health conditions, including medical devices, telemedicine, and health information technology.

19. Patient-centered care - A model of health care delivery that emphasizes the needs and preferences of individual patients, including shared decision-making and care coordination.

20. Population health management - The process of analyzing and improving the health outcomes of entire populations, often through the use of data analytics and coordinated interventions.

21. Public health - The science and practice of protecting and improving the health of communities through disease prevention, health promotion, and health policy.

22. Health promotion - The process of empowering individuals and communities to improve their health and prevent disease through education, behavior change, and community engagement.

23. Disease prevention - The strategies and interventions used to prevent the occurrence or spread of diseases, including immunization, screening, and lifestyle modifications.

24. Health education - The process of providing information and skills to individuals and communities to promote health and prevent disease.

25. Health literacy - The ability

## EXPLANATIONS ON SOME OF THE TOPICS MENTIONED ABOVE

Sure, here is some information on each of the topics you mentioned:

Health care system: The health care system is a complex network of organizations, people, and resources that deliver health care services to meet the health needs of a specific population. It includes hospitals, clinics, physician practices, and other health care facilities, as well as health care professionals, insurance companies, and government agencies.

Health care policy: Health care policy refers to the set of laws, regulations, and guidelines that govern the organization, financing, and delivery of health care services. Health care policy is developed and implemented by government agencies at the federal, state, and local levels, as well as by private organizations and industry groups.

Health care reform: Health care reform is the process of changing and improving the health care system to address deficiencies in access, quality, and affordability. Health care reform can take many forms, including changes to insurance coverage, payment and delivery models, and regulatory frameworks

.

Health care disparities: Health care disparities refer to differences in health outcomes and access to health care services between different populations, often related to social determinants of health such as race, ethnicity, income, and geography. Health care disparities are a major challenge facing the health care system and require targeted interventions to address.

Health care delivery: Health care delivery refers to the process of providing health care services to individuals, including diagnosis, treatment, and management of health conditions. Health care delivery involves a range of health care professionals and facilities, and can take place in a variety of settings, including hospitals, clinics, and home-based care.

Health care quality: Health care quality refers to the degree to which health care services meet established standards of safety, effectiveness, and patient-centeredness. Health care quality is an important measure of the overall performance of the health care system, and efforts to improve quality can lead to better health outcomes and reduced costs.

Health care access: Health care access refers to the ability of individuals to obtain needed health care services. Access to health care services is influenced by a range of factors, including insurance coverage, affordability, and geographic proximity to health care facilities.

Medicaid: Medicaid is a joint federal-state program that provides health insurance coverage for eligible low-income individuals and families. Medicaid is an important source of health care coverage for millions of Americans, and plays a critical role in addressing health care disparities and improving access to care.

Resolution: Resolving health care challenges requires a multi-faceted approach that involves addressing the root causes of health care disparities, improving access to care, and promoting policies that support high-quality, patient-centered care. Resolution requires collaboration between health care providers, policymakers, and communities to identify and implement effective solutions.

Importance: Health care is a critical component of overall well-being, and access to quality health care services is essential for individuals and communities to thrive. Improving the health care system is an important priority for policymakers and health care providers alike, as it has far-reaching implications for both public health and the economy.

Need, Effect and Impact: The need for improved health care is driven by a range of factors, including demographic changes, advances in medical technology, and an increasing burden of chronic disease. The effect of these trends has been to place greater demands on the health care system, and to highlight the need for innovative approaches to health care delivery. The impact of health care challenges can be profound, affecting individuals, families, and communities in a variety of ways. Addressing these challenges requires continued investment in research, policy

## NUTRITIONAL HEALTH

---

Nutritional health refers to the state of an individual's physical, mental, and emotional health as it relates to their nutritional intake. Proper nutritional intake is essential for maintaining optimal health and well-being.

The effects and impact of nutritional health can be seen in several areas of an individual's life, including:

1. Physical health: Adequate nutrition is essential for maintaining a healthy weight, building strong bones and muscles, supporting the immune system, and reducing the risk of chronic diseases such as heart disease, stroke, and diabetes.

2. Mental health: Proper nutrition plays a crucial role in brain function and mental health. Adequate intake of certain nutrients such as omega-3 fatty acids, B vitamins, and magnesium has been linked to a reduced risk of depression and anxiety.

3. Emotional health: Good nutrition can also have a positive impact on emotional health. A balanced diet rich in nutrients such as vitamin C, vitamin E, and beta-carotene has been linked to lower levels of stress and improved mood

.

4. Cognitive function: Nutrition plays a vital role in cognitive function, including memory, attention, and problem-solving ability. Nutrients such as omega-3 fatty acids and B vitamins have been shown to support cognitive function and reduce the risk of cognitive decline.

5. Overall well-being: Proper nutrition is essential for overall well-being. A balanced diet provides the body with the necessary nutrients to function optimally, leading to increased energy levels, Improved sleep, and a greater sense of vitality.

In contrast, poor nutritional health can have negative effects on an individual's health and well-being, including:

1. Increased risk of chronic diseases: A diet high in saturated and trans fats, added sugars, and sodium can increase the risk of chronic diseases such as heart disease, stroke, and diabetes.

2. Decreased cognitive function: Poor nutrition can affect cognitive function, including memory, attention, and problem-solving ability.

3. Increased risk of mental health issues: Inadequate nutrition has been linked to an increased risk of depression and anxiety.

4. Reduced immune function: Poor nutrition can weaken the immune system, making individuals more susceptible to infections and illnesses.

5. Overall decreased quality of life: Poor nutritional health can lead to decreased energy levels, poor sleep, and a general sense of malaise, leading to a reduced quality of life.

In conclusion, proper nutritional health is essential for maintaining optimal health and well-being. A balanced diet rich in essential nutrients can have positive effects on physical, mental, and emotional health, while poor nutritional health can have negative effects on all areas of an individual's life

.

## TYPES AND EXAMPLES

There are several types of nutrients that are essential for good nutritional health. Here are the main types and some examples of each:

1. Carbohydrates: Carbohydrates are the body's primary source of energy. They are found in foods such as grains, fruits, vegetables, and dairy products. Examples of carbohydrates include bread, pasta, rice, cereal, potatoes, bananas, and apples.

2. Proteins: Proteins are essential for building and repairing tissues, as well as for the production of enzymes and hormones. They are found in foods such as meats, poultry, fish, beans, nuts, and dairy products. Examples of proteins include chicken, beef, fish, lentils, almonds, and Greek yogurt.

3. Fats: Fats are important for energy storage, insulation, and protection of organs. They are found in foods such as oils, butter, nuts, and meats. Examples of fats include olive oil, avocado, salmon, and almonds.

4. Vitamins: Vitamins are essential for various bodily functions, including growth, development, and immunity. They are found in fruits, vegetables, and fortified foods. Examples of vitamins include vitamin C (found in citrus

fruits), vitamin A (found in sweet potatoes), and vitamin D (found in fortified milk).

5. Minerals: Minerals are important for strong bones and teeth, as well as for various bodily functions such as muscle contraction and nerve function. They are found in foods such as leafy greens, dairy products, and meats. Examples of minerals include calcium (found in dairy products), iron (found in red meat), and potassium (found in bananas).

6. Water: Water is essential for maintaining hydration and regulating bodily functions. It is found in water, beverages, and some foods such as fruits and vegetables.

In order to maintain good nutritional health, it is important to consume a balanced diet that includes all of these essential nutrients in appropriate amounts.

## THE SIDE EFFECTS OF NOT TAKING THESE FOODS

Not taking adequate amounts of the essential nutrients can lead to various side effects and health problems. Here are some examples:

1. Carbohydrate deficiency: Inadequate carbohydrate intake can lead to low blood sugar levels, fatigue, weakness, dizziness, and headaches. In extreme cases, it can also lead to ketosis, a condition where the body burns fat for energy instead of carbohydrates, which can cause nausea, vomiting, and even coma.

2. Protein deficiency: Inadequate protein intake can lead to muscle wasting, weakness, fatigue, and a weakened immune system. It can also lead to stunted growth and development in children.

3. Fat deficiency: Inadequate fat intake can lead to dry skin, hair loss, and poor wound healing. It can also affect the absorption of fat-soluble vitamins such as vitamin A, D, E, and K.

4. Vitamin deficiency: Inadequate intake of vitamins can lead to various health problems depending on the specific vitamin. For example, vitamin C deficiency can lead to scurvy, which causes bleeding gums, bruising, and fatigue. Vitamin D deficiency can lead to weak bones and increased risk of fractures.

5. Mineral deficiency: Inadequate intake of minerals can lead to various health problems depending on the specific mineral. For example, calcium deficiency can lead to weak bones and increased risk of fractures. Iron deficiency can lead to anemia, which causes fatigue, weakness, and pale skin.

6. Dehydration: Inadequate water intake can lead to dehydration, which can cause fatigue, headache, dizziness, dry mouth and throat, and decreased urine output.

In conclusion, not taking adequate amounts of essential nutrients can lead to various side effects and health problems. It is important to consume a balanced diet that includes all of these essential nutrients in appropriate amounts to maintain good nutritional health and prevent these side effects.

www.ingramcontent.com/pod-product-compliance
Lightning Source LLC
Chambersburg PA
CBHW040316240726

48664CB00006B/1509